Ketosis Diet:
Eat Fat, Be Thin

7 Steps to a Low-Carb Ketosis diet - - Transform your body fast

Disclaimer:

No part of this publication may be reproduced, stored or transmitted in any form or by any means – electronic, mechanical, scanning, photocopying, recording or otherwise, without prior written permission from the author.

This publication is provided for informational and educational purposes only and cannot be used as a substitute for expert medical advice. The information contained herein does not take into account an individual reader's health or medical history.

Hence, it's important to consult with a health care professional before starting any regimen mentioned herein. Though all possible efforts have been made in the preparation of this eBook, the author makes no warranties as to the accuracy or completeness of its contents.

The readers understand that they can follow the information, guidelines and ideas mentioned in this eBook at their own risk. All trademarks mentioned are the property of their respective owners.

Contents

Summary: What to Expect?

Not only will this eBook help you open doors to the subject of ketosis, but also give a comprehensive insight on the mechanics of the ketogenic diet, and how you can incorporate it in your daily to benefit from its multiple perks, including weight-loss.

This eBook is all about tips and tricks, canopying everything concerning a healthy and effective weight loss regimen.

INTRODUCTION: WHAT IS KETOSIS?

Firstly, the word ketosis refers to the state of the human body when it lacks carbohydrates and starts depending upon proteins, fat and muscle for its energy. That is how this diet got its name. In other words, a ketosis diet is a diet with low amount of carbs or no carbs at all.

Being in this condition, the brain tells your body to create reserves of glucose for emergencies only. This happens because of the lack of carbohydrates in your body. And so, the brain starts using fat storages for immediate energy needs.

When you first deprive your body of carbohydrates and replace them with protein and fat, the metabolism shifts to accommodate this. The first stage is known as lipolysis, and is the initial burning of fat to use as energy.

Ketosis is the second part of the process that takes place when your body's metabolism shifts from getting energy from carbohydrates to taking it from fat. When it is taking place, this is the time you lose the most fat. The term **ketosis** relates to the blocks of fat that are stored for release as energy, which are known as ketones.

HISTORY OF THE KETOSIS DIET

Epilepsy has confounded humanity since its earliest manifestations in the individuals it plagued. Once attributed to supernatural attacks from evil spirits, the disease soon came under the scrutiny of Hippocrates. The Greek were the first to identify the reality of Epilepsy being biological and not spiritual. It was Hippocrates who would use fasting as a means of correcting the disease.

But Hippocrates wasn't alone. As history unfolded after Hippocrates, other physicians cited fasting as a means for combating Epilepsy. This is what makes the Ketogenic Diet so incredible: it has been developed over centuries of time, and the physicians who were working to find a cure had no idea! Fortunately for the world, they were on the right track, and this track would lead to the Ketogenic Diet breakthrough of the 20th century.

Early in the 20th century, there was a worldwide interest in fasting as a means of treating epilepsy. It peaked when two doctors (Guelpa & Marie) from Paris helped 20 people minimize the effects of their epilepsy and recorded the entire process in a report.

Soon after, the same conclusions were drawn in the US when doctors from multiple fields used fasting to improve their patients' situations. But we know that while fasting is a temporary cure, it's unsustainable.

FROM FASTING TO THE KETOGENIC DIET:

To understand the transition from fasting to dieting, it's important to see the connection made by William Lennox of the Harvard Medical School. He observed that seizures began to subside after 2 – 3 days of fasting, which led him to conclude that the change came from a change in metabolism, more specifically, a change in the body's fuel.

The body began fueling itself on fat, Lennox suggested. The connection of fat as fuel in the fasting subjects was paramount in the development of the Ketogenic Diet.

In 1921, the endocrinologist, Dr. Rollin Woodyatt, discovered that acetone and beta-hydroxybutyric were present in people who followed a fast or a certain diet that was low in carbs and high in fats.

Keep in mind that acetone and beta-hydroxybutyric are members of the Ketone family. This had a huge impact on

Dr. Russell Wilder, who would make another discovery the same year.

Dr. Wilder realized that though fasting was effective, it wasn't sustainable. Wilder proposed that the body could produce the same ketone bodies that it produced during fasting, except with the patient eating regularly. This prolonged state of Ketonemia would be what Wilder termed the Ketogenic Diet.

Dr. Wilder's discovery of the Ketogenic Diet blew open the doors for innovation! Dr. Peterman, a physician at the Mayo Clinic, was the first to standardize the diet by developing the following calculations:

– 1g of protein per kilogram of bodyweight

– 10 – 15 g of carbs per day

– Fill the rest of the remaining calories with fat

Aside from some mild alterations to the diet, this is basically the same diet practiced today! With Dr. Peterman's metrics guiding them, other doctors began experimenting with this wonderful new diet that was a godsend for people struggling with epilepsy.

Dr. Peterman also noticed the effects of the Ketogenic Diet on the brain's performance, noting that people adhering to the Ketogenic diet displayed "a marked change in character, concomitant with the ketosis, a decrease in irritability, and an increased interest and alertness."

The Ketogenic Diet was impacting the most important parts of the body and science had finally caught up to document the incredible exchange. The Ketogenic Diet became the unquestioned best weapon in the fight against epilepsy. The diet was so effective in fact, that it has been in competition with the pharmaceutical industry since 1938, when the first antiepileptic drugs hit the market.

The next thirty years were bleak for the Ketogenic Diet. Antiepileptic drugs offered epilepsy patients a way around seizures without having to adhere to a strict diet. It seems like many at the time chalked the diet up to be archaic, used in the time it was pragmatic for, and then retired when something better came along. But there were still those who wanted to prove the worthiness of the Ketogenic Diet.

In 1971, an easier to follow Medium-Chain Triglyceride oil diet was developed in hopes of getting people who were on the fence about the diet to give it a shot, but this attempt proved futile. The problem was that the diet was viewed as beneficial only for epilepsy patients. Few thought it could be utilized for other dieting purposes. People had yet to realize the Ketogenic Diet was useful for so much more than treating epilepsy, although that was a massive benefit.

Years passed with little to no development on the Ketogenic Diet. Antiepileptic drugs ruled the field. That was until a reality shaking episode of *Dateline* was produced in 1994. Dateline followed a tormented boy named Charlie Abrahams, who had suffered from what seemed like endless seizures for the first two years of his life. His parents tried everything: faith healing, antiepileptics, homeopathic medicine, and even brain surgery. The diagnosis looked grim for poor Charlie.

That was until Charlie's father, Jim Abrahams, discovered the Ketogenic Diet while researching treatments for epilepsy. Charlie was taken to Johns Hopkins where he began the diet and saw immediate results. Not only was Charlie able to control his seizures, but he also made significant cognitive development that was previously thought unlikely by his doctors. Charlie's father was confounded. Why hadn't anyone told them sooner about the diet and its benefits for children with epilepsy?

Realizing that other families could be going through the same thing, Jim took action. He started the Charlie Foundation and began producing resources for other families who were in the fight against epilepsy. The Abrahams could have never known how important their work was going to be. The fact that they managed to bring the spotlight back to the Ketogenic Diet and its efficacy for treating epilepsy has reinvigorated interest in the diet.

The Ketogenic Diet's origins are founded in the pursuit of scientific truth. It is a remedy based on the principle of helping and healing, not making money or creating addicts. Keep pursuing the Keto lifestyle, and show everyone around just how powerful this diet is!

SEVEN LOW-CARB LIVING TIPS
FOR WEIGHT LOSS

The low-carb eating in the form of ketosis has a positive effect on hormone regulation-also known as blood sugar regulation, acts a fat burning furnace, and brings the body a number of benefits. Here are seven tips for low-carb living that can help you lose weight... and keep the weight off!

1. Avoid Sugar and Starch

Sugar and starch are a form of carbohydrates, which if consumed in excess, will turn into fat as our liver has no choice to turn that energy into fat and that liver fat leads to further metabolic diseases. Start by limiting your carbohydrate intake to 20 grams a day by avoiding carb-rich foods like flour, pasta, sugar, rice and starchy vegetables. Go through nutrient labels on the consumables and keep a track of your daily carb consumption.

2. Eat "Real Foods"

Medium chain triglycerides (MCT) foods, such as coconut oil, yogurt, and butter consist of good fats, and are easily broken down and used as energy. Highly absorbent, MCTs are commonly used as a therapeutic treatment for malabsorption related issues, including Crohn's Disease. MCTs have also shown benefits when used by people who don't have a gallbladder.

3. Eat Fat to Lose Fat

Although you shouldn't limit yourself to eating meager quantities of oils and butter, you shouldn't consume more once you start feeling full.

4. Eat Greens Every Day

Vegetables are rich with minerals otherwise hard to obtain, like magnesium, potassium, calcium, manganese, folate and betain. The fiber content also speeds up bowel movements, preventing stomach problems while giving the body an overall healthy, refreshing boost. The best way to eat more greens is eating a cup of non-starchy vegetables, raw, and 2 cups of salad greens.

Veggies can include broccoli, summer squash, wax beans, zucchini, jicama, mushrooms, asparagus, Brussels sprouts, leeks, cucumber, egg plant, shallots, rhubarb, celery artichokes, peppers, okra, tomatoes, and pumpkins. It should be remembered that certain vegetables contain a significant amount of carbs, and so should be zigzagged with good fats in your diet.

5. Drink Lots of Liquids

Besides dehydrating yourself with a minimum of 2 liters (at least 8 glasses) of water, drink bouillon to lessen fatigue and headache (unless you are hypertensive). Have a can of caffeinated diet soda or up to 3 cups of coffee a day.

6. Increase Activity While Reducing Stress:

Inactive muscles and a stressed mind can go a long way towards impacting the body negatively and making weight loss much harder. Stress may also lead to excessive dietary temptations, like sugar cravings. Increasing the daily activity will keep your mind occupied and manage your sweet tooth while decreasing appetite, building muscle and improving bone density.

7. Eat When You're Hungry, Stop When You're Full

It is great to start off by knowing the difference between hunger and cravings. If you are moderately hungry, feed your body the essential foods so you don't end up wanting more and overeating. If you've had your fair share of food, but are still tempted to eat, distract yourself with activities.

Listen to your body... if you're not hungry you don't have to eat. Even when you eat, make sure you eat until you are not feeling hungry, NOT until you're full. It's better to satiate your hunger 80%, while leaving the 20% intact.

KETOGENIC DIET PLAN

For the best diet to rapidly burn fat using the body's natural metabolism, consider the ketogenic diet plan. Nutrition has the strongest effect on the body's production of important hormones, which regulate metabolism and allow the body to burn fat for energy and retain muscle mass, with little need for excessive exercise.

WHAT IS A KETOGENIC DIET PLAN?

Basically, it is a diet that causes the body to enter a state of ketosis. Ketosis is a natural and healthy metabolic state in which the body burns its own stored fat (producing ketones), instead of using glucose (the sugars from carbohydrates found in the standard American diet - SAD).

Metabolically speaking, ketogenic foods are powerful. The amazing benefit is these foods are also delicious, natural whole foods that are extremely healthy for you.

SO, WHICH FOODS ARE ENCOURAGED?

Some of the best-tasting, most fulfilling foods are part of this plan, including lean meats like chicken and beef, healthy sources of protein and high-quality fats like avocado, eggs, coconut oil, butter, eggs and olive oil. Also, delicious leafy-green vegetables like kale, chard, and spinach, as well as cruciferous vegetables like broccoli, cabbage and cauliflower.

These foods can be combined with nuts, seeds and sprouts, and a wide range of other amazing foods that lead to incredible health benefits that give your body the protein, healthy fats, and nutrients it needs while providing metabolism-boosting meals for easy cooking at home or on the go.

WHICH FOODS SHOULD BE LIMITED?

On a ketogenic diet plan, the main foods to avoid are those high in carbohydrates, sugars, and the wrong types of fats. These foods can be toxic to the body and create excess glucose that the body turns into stored fat.

These foods increase the level of insulin and blood sugar in the body, and will prevent fat loss even if you are putting a lot of energy into exercise. To avoid these foods, limit your intake of grains, processed foods, vegetable oils (canola, corn, soybean, etc.), milk, margarine, and other high-carbohydrate, high-sugar foods.

BUT AREN'T FATS BAD FOR YOU?

We have been told for decades that calories from fats should be reduced to encourage weight loss, but this is a vast over-simplification (still supported by government and industrial food interests) that is no longer accurate according our modern understanding of human nutrition.

The reality is that certain fats are not good for you (omega-6 fatty acids), because your body has a hard time processing them. Other fats, particularly medium chain triglycerides (MCTs), are extremely beneficial for weight loss, brain cell generation, and nutrients. These healthy saturated fats should be increased to give your body the energy it needs while in ketosis, while limiting the detrimental trans-fats found in many processed foods.

BENEFITS OF THE KETOGENIC DIET

The list of benefits concerning a ketogenic diet is a lengthy and happy one. These are some of the perks of the diet you can expect to see after a month of switching to the ketogenic diet plan:

1- Being in ketosis allows the body to process fat and use it as fuel. Carbohydrates are much easier to convert and use as fuel, so when you are providing plenty of these to your body, you need to burn and use all of it before your body will finally begin converting and using fat as fuel!

2 - Another benefit of being in a state of ketosis is that excess ketones are not harmful to your system in any way whatsoever. Any ketones the body produces, which are not needed are simply excreted through urine, easily and harmlessly. In fact, this excellent benefit is the reason why you can check whether you are in a state of ketosis using urine testing strips in the morning.

3- When your body gets used to being in ketosis, it will actually begin to prefer ketones to glucose. This is the ideal state you want your body to be in: no longer craving sugar whatsoever, and in fact preferring protein as a fuel source as opposed to sugar.

4- Another benefit of the ketogenic diet weight loss is that being in a ketogenic state is useful for controlling insulin levels in the body. Insulin is one of the substances that make you crave food, particularly because it is high in sugar, and so controlling it at healthy levels is one of the key elements of weight loss.

5- Most research studies on the benefits of ketosis diets for epileptic seizures in children show a large improvement, which is especially significant since these children usually did not respond to previous medication therapy. In one study, 38% of the kids on the ketosis diet had more than a 50% reduction in the frequency of seizures while 7% had greater than a 90% reduction. A modified Atkins diet, basically an extended Atkins induction phase, showed similar results.

6- Last, but certainly not least, is that a majority of people who take advantage of ketogenic diet weight loss report that being in a ketogenic state makes them feel significantly less hungry than when they are in a non-ketogenic state. It is much easier to stick to a diet, any diet, when you're not fighting cravings and hunger every step of the way. In fact, hunger pangs can often derail a person's best efforts! Not having to deal with them makes it easier to meet your goals, all the way around.

MAKING THE KETOGETIC DIETS WORK

The Truth

Ketogenic Diets (more specifically Cyclic Ketogenic Diets) are most effective for achieving rapid, ultra low body fat levels with maximum muscle retention! Now, as with all such general statements, there are circumstantial exceptions. But done right, which they rarely are, the fat loss achievable on a ketogenic diet is nothing short of staggering! And, despite what people might tell you, you will also enjoy incredible high energy and overall sense of wellbeing.

The Perception

Despite these promises, more bodybuilders/shapers have had negative experiences than having seen positive results. The main criticisms are:

- Chronic lethargy
- Unbearable hunger
- Massive decrease in gym performance
- Severe muscle loss

All these criticisms result from a failure to heed the caveat: Ketogenic Diets must be done right! It must be realized they are an entirely unique metabolic modality that adheres to none of the previously accepted 'rules' of dieting. And there is no going half-way; 50 grams of carbohydrates per day plus high protein intake is NOT ketogenic!

So, how are ketogenic diets 'done right'? Let's quickly look at how they work.

OVERVIEW OF KETOSIS:

Simply, our body, organs, muscles and brain can use either glucose or ketones for fuel. It is the function of the liver and pancreas (primarily) to regulate that fuel supply and they show a strong bias toward sticking with glucose.

Glucose is the 'preferred' fuel because it is derived in abundance from the diet and readily available readily from liver and muscle stores. Ketones have to be deliberately synthesized by the liver, but the liver can easily synthesize glucose (a process known as 'gluconeogenesis' that uses amino acids (protein) or other metabolic intermediaries) too.

We don't get beta hydroxybutyrate, acetone, or acetoacetate (ketones) from the diet. The liver synthesizes them only under duress, as a last measure in conditions of severe glucose deprivation, like starvation. For the liver to be convinced that ketones are the order of the day, several conditions must be met:

- Blood glucose must fall below 50mg/dl
- Low blood glucose must result in low Insulin and elevated Glucagon
- Liver glycogen must be low or 'empty'
- A plentiful supply of gluconeogenic substrates must NOT be available

At this point, it is important to mention that it is not actually a question of being 'in' or 'out' of ketosis. We don't either totally run on ketones, or not. It is a gradual and careful transition so that the brain is constantly and evenly fuelled... ideally. Ketones SHOULD be produced in small amounts from blood glucose levels of about 60mg/dl. We consider ourselves in ketosis when there are greater concentrations of ketones than glucose in the blood.

The reality is that most people, especially weight trainers, have had a regular intake of glucose for a good couple of decades, at least. The liver is perfectly capable of producing ketones but the highly efficient gluconeogenic pathways are able to maintain low-normal blood glucose above the ketogenic threshold.

Couple this with the fact that many people are at least partially insulin resistant and have elevated fasting insulin (upper end of the normal range, anyway). The small amount of blood glucose from gluconeogenesis induces sufficient insulin release to blunt glucagon output and the production of ketones.

Sudden glucose deprivation will cause, initially, lethargy, hunger, and weakness, in most people, until ketosis is achieved. And Ketosis will not be reached until the liver is forced to quit with gluconeogenesis and start producing ketones. As long as dietary protein is sufficient, the liver will continue to produce glucose and not ketones. That's why no carb, high protein diets are NOT ketogenic.

What Is So Great About Ketosis Anyway?

When the body switches over to running primarily on ketones, a number of cool things happen:

-Lipolysis (bodyfat breakdown) is substantially increased

-Muscle catabolism (muscle loss) is substantially reduced

-Energy levels are maintained in a high and stable state

-Subcutaneous fluid (aka 'water retention') is eliminated

Basically, when we are in ketosis our body is using fat (ketones) to fuel everything. As such, we aren't breaking down muscle to provide glucose. That is, muscle is being spared because it has nothing to offer. Fat is all the body needs (well, to a large extent). For the dieter, this means substantially less muscle loss than what is achievable on any other diet. Makes sense?

As a bonus, ketones yield only 7 calories per gram. This is higher than the equal mass of glucose but substantially less (22%, in fact) than the 9 calories per gram of fat from whence it came. We like metabolic inefficiencies like this. They mean we can eat more but the body doesn't get the calories.

Even cooler is that ketones cannot be turned back into fatty acids. The body excretes any excess in the urine! Speaking of which, there will be quite a bit of urine. The drop in muscle glycogen, low Insulin and low aldosterone all equate to massive excretion of intra and extracellular fluid. For us that means hard, defined muscularity and quick visible results.

Regarding energy, our brain actually really likes ketones so we tend to feel fantastic in ketosis: clearheaded, alert and positive. And because there is never a shortage of fat to supply ketones, energy is high all the time. Usually you even sleep less than usual and wake up feeling more refreshed when in ketosis.

DOING IT RIGHT:

From what is said above, you will notice that to get into ketosis:

- Carbohydrate intake should be nil; Zero!
- Protein intake should be low - 25% of calories at a maximum
- Fat must account for 75%+ of calories

With low insulin (due to zero carbs) and calories at, or below maintenance, the dietary fat cannot be deposited in adipose tissues. The low-ish protein means that gluconeogenesis will quickly prove inadequate to maintain blood glucose and, whether the body likes it or not, there is still all the damned fat to burn.

And burn it does. The high dietary fat is oxidized for cellular energy in the normal fashion but winds up generating quantities of Acetyl-CoA that exceed the capacity of the TCA cycle. The significant result is ketogenesis, synthesis of ketones from the excess Acetyl-CoA. In more lay terms: the high fat intake "forces" ketosis upon the body. This is how it's done right.

Now you just have to throw out what you thought was true about fats. Firstly, fat does not "make you fat". Most of the information about the evils of saturated fats, in particular, is so disproportionate or plain wrong anyway. On a ketogenic diet, it is doubly inapplicable. Saturated fats make ketosis fly. And don't worry, your heart will be better than fine and your insulin sensitivity will NOT be reduced (there is no insulin around in the first place)!

Once in ketosis it is not necessary, technically speaking, to maintain absolute zero carbs or low protein. But it is still better if you want to reap the greatest rewards. Besides, assuming you are training hard, you will still want to follow a cyclic ketogenic diet where you get to eat all your carbs, fruit and whatever else, every 1-2 weeks, anyway (more on this in another article).

Don't be mistaken: 'done right' does not make ketogenic dieting easy or fun for the culinary acrobats among you. They are probably the most restrictive diets you can use and not an option if you don't love animal products. Get out your nutritional almanac and work out an 20:0:80 protein: carb: fat diet. Yeah, it's boring. As an example, your writer's daily ketogenic diet is 3100 Calories at 25:0.5:74.5 from only:

- 10 XXL Whole Eggs
- 160ml Pure Cream (40% fat)
- 400g Mince (15% fat)
- 60ml Flaxseed Oil
- 30g Whey Protein Isolate

Supplementation:

There are a number of supplements that assist in making Ketogenic diets more effective. However, many popular supplements would be wasted. Here is an overview of the main ones:

- Chromium and ALA, while not insulin 'mimickers' as many claim, increase insulin sensitivity, resulting in lower insulin levels, higher glucagon and a faster descent into deeper ketosis

- Creatine is a bit of a waste - at most, 30% can be taken up by the muscles that, without glycogen, cannot be meaningfully 'volumized'.

- HMB (if it works) would/should be an excellent supplement for minimizing the catabolic period before ketosis is achieved

- Tribulus is excellent and comes highly recommended as it magnifies the increased testosterone output of a ketogenic diet

- Carnitine in L or Acetyl-L form is an essential supplement for Ketogenic Diets. L-Carnitine is necessary for the formation of Ketones in the liver.

- Glutamine, free-form essential and branched-chain aminos are worthwhile for pre and post training. Just don't overdo the glutamine as it supports gluconeogenesis

- ECA stack fat burners are useful and important though don't worry about the inclusion of HCA

- Flaxseed oil is great but do not think that you need 50% of your calories from essential fatty acids. 1-10% of calories are more than sufficient.

- Whey Protein is optional - you don't want too much protein remember

- A soluble fiber supplement that is non-carbohydrate based is good. But walnuts are easier.

Ketogenic diets offer a host of unique benefits that cannot be ignored if you are chasing the ultimate, low body-fat figure or physique. However, they are not the most user- friendly of diets and any 'middle ground' compromise you might prefer will be just the worst of all worlds. Your choice is to do them right or not at all.

FIVE TIPS

FOR SUCCESS ON THE KETOGENIC DIET

Just getting started on the ketogenic diet? Good for you! Following are some of the important hacks to remember when following your diet plan in order to get the most out of it, and maximize your success rate.

1. HYDRATE YOURSELF

Your body finds it difficult to retain water when on a ketogenic diet, so replenishing your body with plenty of fluids, especially water is crucial. Drink a minimum of three liters of water a day, and take your urine color as an indicator of proper hydration. A gentle yellow means you are properly hydrated.

2. REMEMBER THE FATS

Our bodies need fuel to function. When we restrict our carbs intake, especially to the point where it activates ketosis, back-up fuel is needed by our bodies. Because protein is not a great source of energy, fat is the option our bodies turn to.

The good news is that while in ketosis, most of the fat eaten is turned into energy, and not stored. Therefore, it is important that you choose a wide variety of unsaturated, healthy fat containing foods, like nuts, avocados, dairy products, olives and seeds for consumption.

3. BE SMART ABOUT LIQUOR

Another great perk of the ketosis diet is the ability to enjoy alcohol without compromising your weight loss efforts. Try switching to unsweetened drinks, like scotch, whiskey, vodka, tequila, rum, gin, brandy and cognac while occasionally treating yourself to a low-carb beer.

Low-carb mixers should be your choice of drink, and remember to stay fully hydrated as hangovers are especially bad while in ketosis. Remember to not go crazy as calories still count.

4. BE PATIENT

Remember that weight loss is not an overnight process, and so don't freak out or lose motivation, and stop weighing yourself every other day! The results are gradual and require persistence and a strong willpower.

TEN LOW-CARB DIET MYTHS DEBUNKED

Before jumping into anything new, we all have questions. If you are curious, and looking for answers regarding the authenticity of myths that soar about low-carb diets, like ketosis, now is the chance to educate yourself. Here we have compiled a list of the10 most popular myths concerning low-carb diets, and the truth behind these statements.

Myth #1:

The low-carb diet is dangerous. The truth is that it is not, and has been proven over the years to be safe and extremely effective. Dr. Atkins gets credit for this diet, but he was not even close to being the innovator, he just brought it into the mainstream, which brings us to myth #2.

Myth #2:

The truth is the father of low-carb, high protein diet dates back to 1863. William Banting of England who wrote a little booklet titled "Letter on Corpulence Addressed to the Public" is considered the father of low carbohydrate dieting. He proved this over years, helping people lose weight without any side effects.

Myth #3:

Low-carbs, high protein and high fat raises cholesterol. The truth behind this statement is it actually lowers cholesterol. For one year, researchers at the Veterans Affairs Medical Center in Philadelphia followed 132 obese adults randomized into two groups.

The carb intake for one group was below 30 grams a day, while for the other, their overall daily caloric intake was reduced by 500 calories with 30% of the calories coming from fat sources. 83% of the study group had diabetes or other risk factors for heart disease.

In the low-carb group, triglyceride levels decreased more and HDL ('good') cholesterol levels decreased less than in the low-fat group. (High levels of triglycerides, a fat in the blood, are associated with heart disease.) People with diabetes on the low-carb diet had better control of blood sugar.

Another research study, published in the Annals of Internal Medicine, involved 120 overweight people and was conducted over a period of six months. Researchers from the Duke University found that participants on the low-carb diet lost 26 pounds, on average, whereas the other group averaged 14 pounds.

The low-carbohydrate group had more beneficial changes in blood triglyceride levels and HDL cholesterol levels than the low-fat diet group. In this study, the low-carb diet groups also received vitamins and other nutritional supplements.

Myth #4:

The low carb diet will cause my blood pressure to rise. Again, the truth is with lower LDL levels and VLDL levels, blood pressure levels actually drop. Lead author, Dr. William S. Yancy Jr, associate professor of medicine at Duke, said their findings send an important message to people with high blood pressure who are trying to lose weight.

Myth #5:

You need carbohydrates or glucose for your brain to function. The truth is if you are on a hardcore low-carb high protein diet, where carbohydrates are non-existent, you are on what is called a Ketogenic Diet. When on a strict diet, your body produces ketones in the absence of carbohydrates, and then converts the ketones into a form of glucose that enables proper brain function. This brings us to the next myth.

Myth #6:

You cannot eat any carbs on a high protein diet. Using the Atkins diet as an example, Atkins himself said on the Larry King show, "You can eat all the carbs your body allows as long as you do not gain weight". What he was talking about was when we reach our desired weight you can add as many carbs to your diet until you start gaining weight, that is your threshold, for some people it is 50 grams a day for others it's 200 grams or more.

Myth #7:

I will gain all my weight back if I stop my low carb diet. This is totally false. It does not matter which diet you choose, if you are successful in your weight loss and then stop your diet, 9 out of 10 times you revert back to your old eating habits, and start eating junk and overindulge, then of course you gain weight back.

Myth #8:

Eating protein makes you fat. This statement doesn't hold much truth. Protein actually raises your calorie burning metabolism by as much as 30% over carbohydrates. When proteins are consumed, your body must digest and break them down into amino acids. This takes energy and plenty of it, which actually helps you lose weight, not gain it.

Myth #9:

High protein diets include fats, and fats are bad for me. Fats in the absence of carbohydrates burn more efficiently, and do not clog your arteries. As the studies show LDL levels (low density lipoproteins) which are the artery cloggers, are lowered. The levels of HDLs, which are the good triglycerides are raised even though your fat intake is increased, that as mentioned above is attributed to low carb intake.

As is previously mentioned, carbs and fat don't mix, and your body cannot efficiently break them down together. Your liver is overburdened and ends up converting the carbohydrates into fat, unless of course you are exercising like crazy.

Myth #10:

I will not have any energy with the low carb diet. This statement is totally false, unless you are a marathon runner or bodybuilder. When you consume small amounts of carbohydrates, your body needs another source of energy. When glycogen levels are gone, your body starts using fat for energy and combustion.

If you are extremely active, it will take about 2-3 weeks, after which your body is acclimated to your new eating habits and adjusts, energizing you as before. If you are involved in an endurance sport, then of course you need extra carbs to be competitive. If you are an athlete or workout extensively, you probably would not be dieting anyway, and a low carb high carb is a moot point.

Conclusion

With this, we come to the end of our eBook on the Ketosis Diet. Over the course of the eBook, we have covered all the information you will need to start following the Ketosis Diet and also achieve success with it.

As long as you stick to the information provided here and follow the tips, you shouldn't have any problem shedding the extra pounds in no time. It is truly the best approach to losing weight fast, but in a healthy and safe manner.

www.ingramcontent.com/pod-product-compliance
Lightning Source LLC
Chambersburg PA
CBHW072020290526
45787CB00013B/1523